Eternal and Soul
Have Forever

A Story of Love, Loss, Recovery, and Redemption

MARY ANNE
HOWARD-CLARKE, RN, RM

BALBOA.PRESS

A DIVISION OF HAY HOUSE

Balboa Press books may be ordered through booksellers or by contacting:

Balboa Press
A Division of Hay House
1663 Liberty Drive
Bloomington, IN 47403
www.balboapress.com.au
1 (877) 407-4847

Print information available on the last page.

ISBN: 978-1-5043-2104-4 (sc)
ISBN: 978-1-5043-2105-1 (e)

Balboa Press rev. date: 05/28/2020

Contents

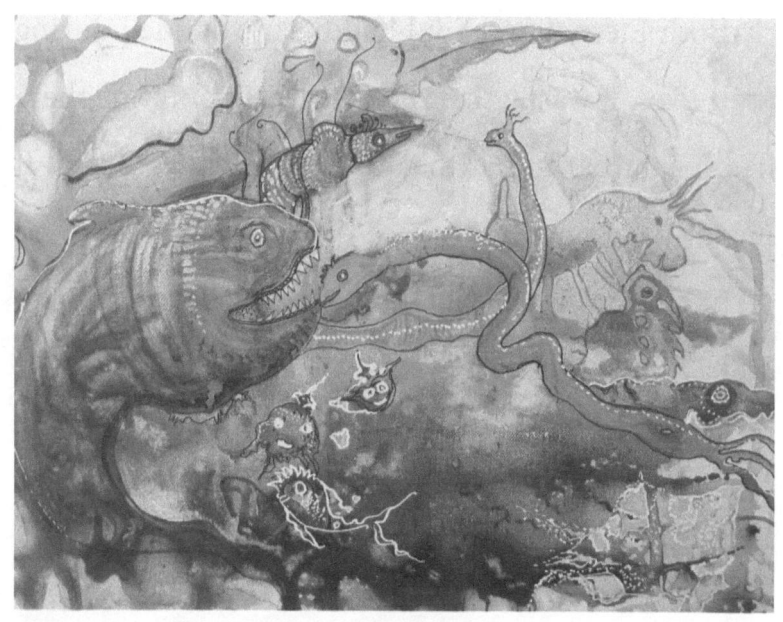

Once upon a time, on a planet called Earth, there lived two people, Eternal and Soul.

They were very excited as they had just discovered that they were to have the most wonderful experience. Forever had chosen them to be its parents and was growing inside Eternal's body.

Eternal and Soul were both so happy. They realised that they wanted Forever to be the most amazing person and to have the most wonderful life possible.

How could they help that happen?

Both Eternal and Soul had been wounded during their lives. It wasn't that the people surrounding them had meant harm, but they too had been wounded. It meant that sometimes these people chose to say and do hurtful things, although they were just reacting to and acting out of past events.

I love myself.

People in my life love and respect me.

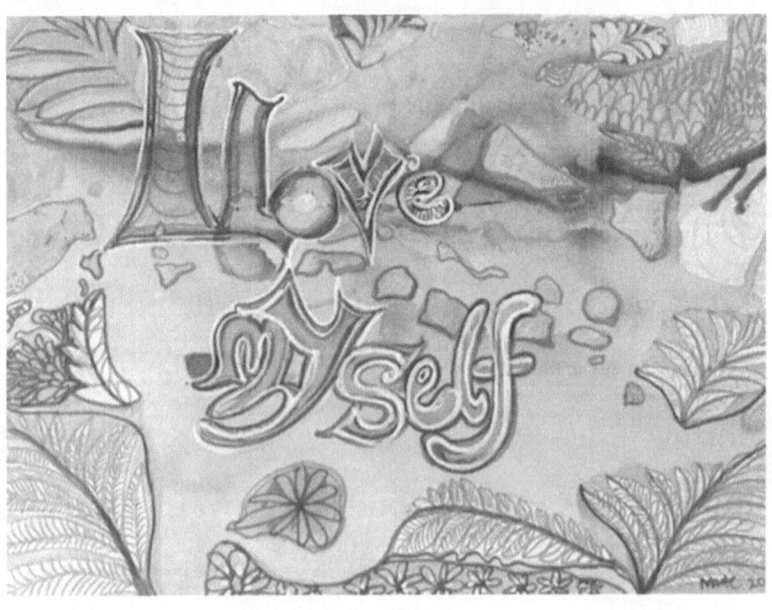

Chapter 1

Eternal's mother was an alcoholic, and her father was abusive. Eternal had been so wounded during her early life that she chose never to feel or think about the awful words that her mother said to her or the terrible physical abuse her father inflicted on her or the pain that her sister's demeaning words caused her. So day after day, her body was flooded with this vile stuff, and it often caused her to say and do hurtful things to others. And yet the next day, she was often unable to remember any of the words or the pain she caused.

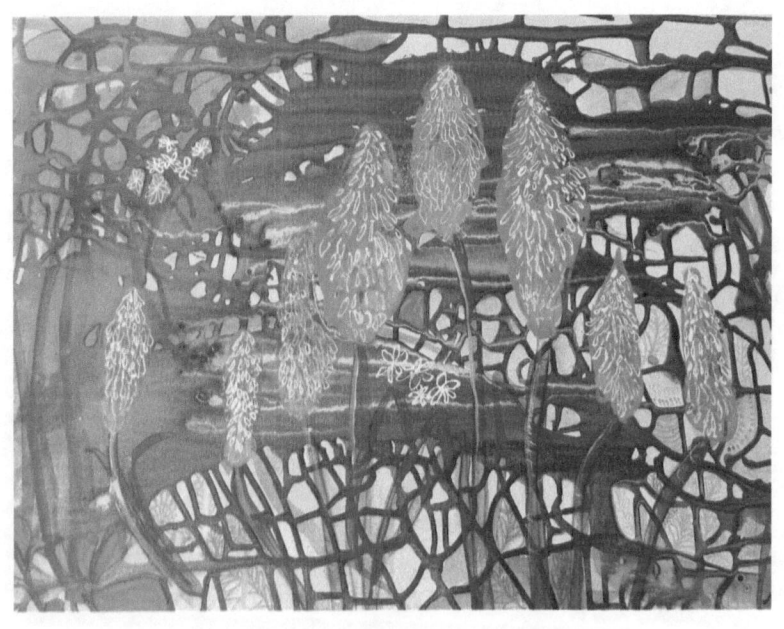

Everyone in my life loves and respects me.

Chapter 2

Wounding self-talk was so often reflected in Eternal's life that she was unconsciously sabotaging every part of her life. Her mother's words were recalled over and over again. They pierced her like sharp arrows, and she believed that it was all her fault! She was useless, lazy, emotional, and dumb, so she had begun to loathe herself internally. Gradually—so gradually she did not really notice it—she was saying the most terrible things to herself all the time.

Eternal's life became very hard. It seemed that the things she told herself were all coming true.

How she wasn't good at things, that no one liked her, and she was always left out. Her friends and even Soul treated her badly. She started to choose a lifestyle that wasn't good or life affirming because she just didn't care.

Eternal knew that beneath it all, her mother had been a good person and the best mother that she was able to be. But the damage had been done.

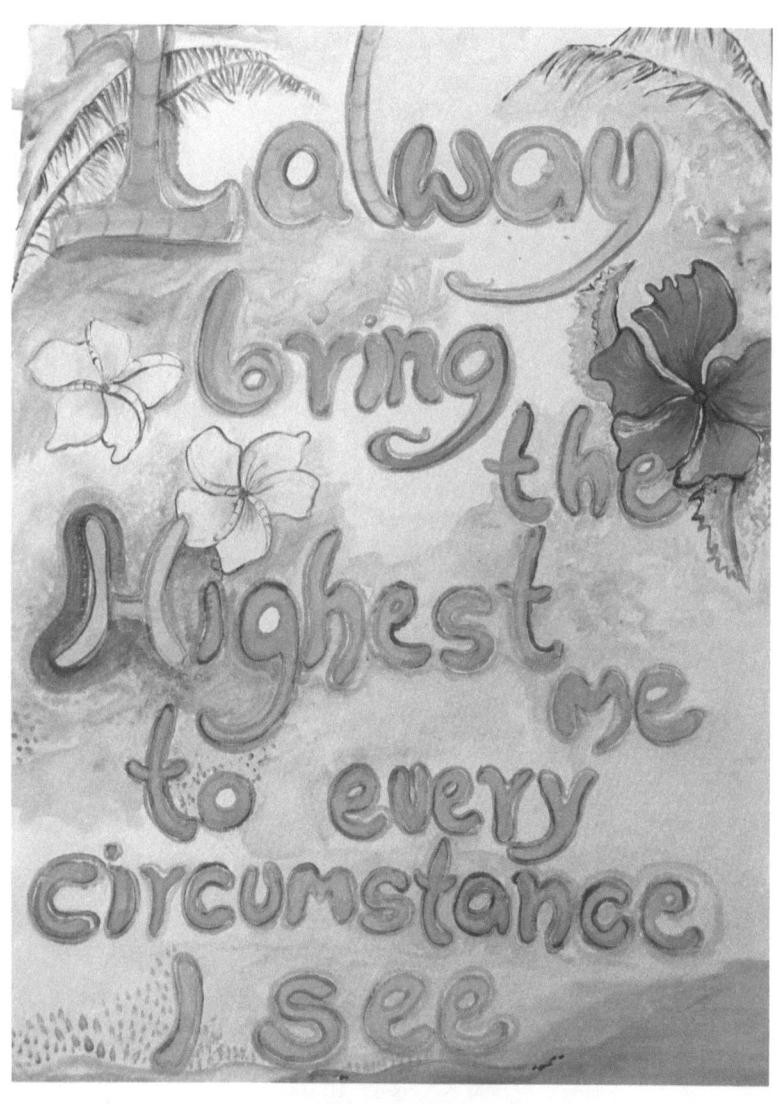

I alway bring the Highest me to every circumstance I see

I love and forgive every person who has been part of my life.

Chapter 3

Soul was also wounded. He had been born into a poor family. Soul was so ashamed of his circumstances, his early environment, and the strata of life he had been born into that he chose to live his life doing not what he wanted to do but only work designed to bring him significant wealth to ensure he would never have to feel the shame of his poor background again.

He achieved wealth, but sadly, his terrible fear of poverty and losing everything, and his obsession with his humble upbringing, affected his reality. He would achieve wealth only to lose it again and again.

Then, in his pain and inward focus, which manifested often as anger, he would unconsciously wound Eternal. Soul knew that beneath it all, his father had been a good person and, despite his poor circumstances, the best father he knew how to be.

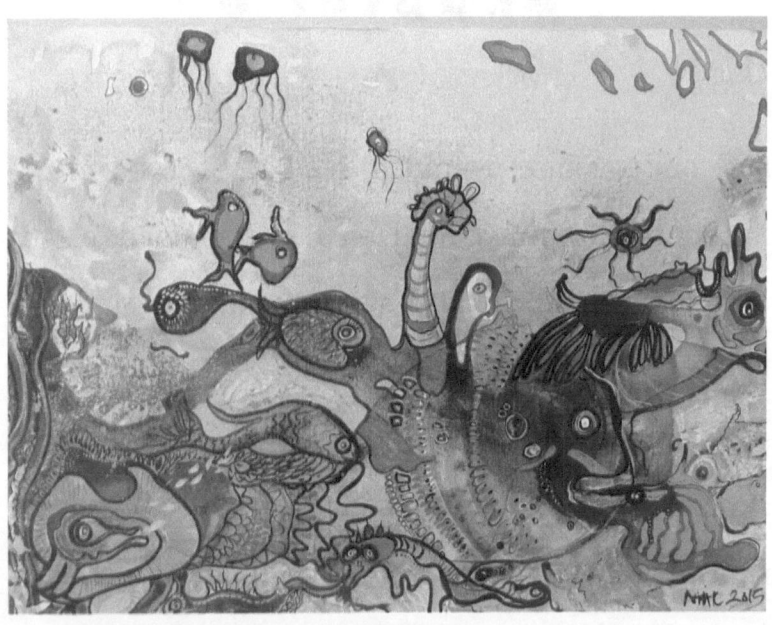

Abundance in all ways is irresistibly drawn to me.

Chapter 4

Eternal and Soul made a pact to change their lives and to become the best parents possible. They were so inspired and excited at Forever growing quietly in Eternal.

Wonderful things—people, books, events—started appearing in their lives. Eternal and Soul met Thoughts, and he made them realise that everything we think and say to ourselves becomes our reality.

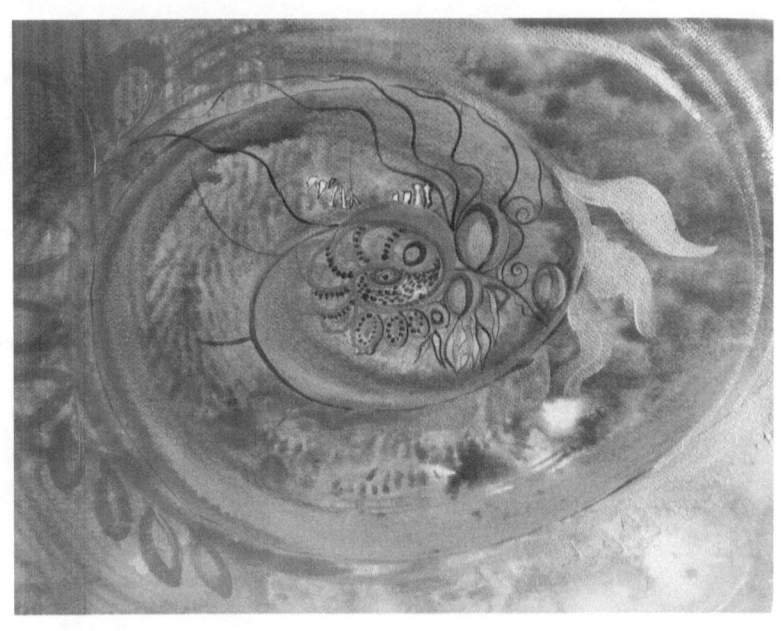

You are what you think.

We are all subject to the law of our own consciousness.

Take care of your own thoughts.

Eternal and Soul decided to think only the highest thoughts they could and replace their wounded old thoughts with new positive ones.

In conversations with friends, Eternal noticed that many, if not most people were unable to love themselves. It was all part of humanity's affliction.

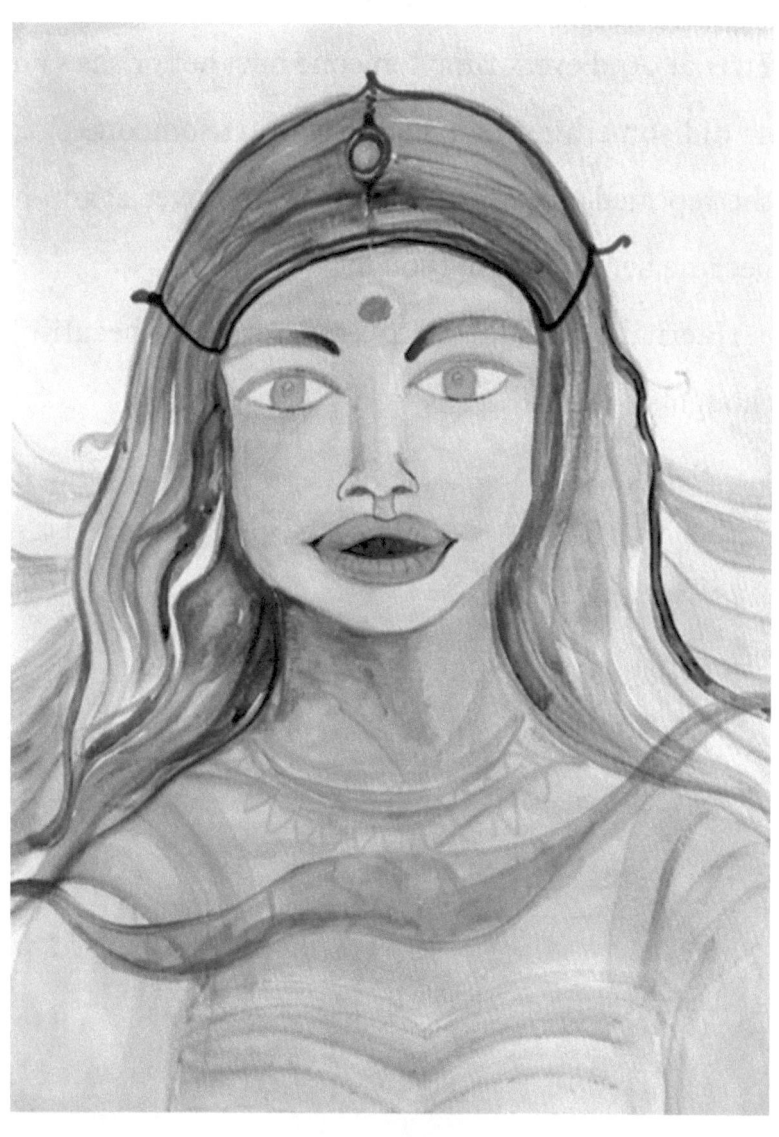

I love myself, I love myself, I love myself.

I am love, I am love, I am love.

This became the most soothing mantra for Eternal. And every time someone hurt her or she said or did something that she knew hurt someone else, she repeated this affirmation over and over again. It became her dominant thought.

Eternal and Soul discovered so many beautiful thoughts, such as

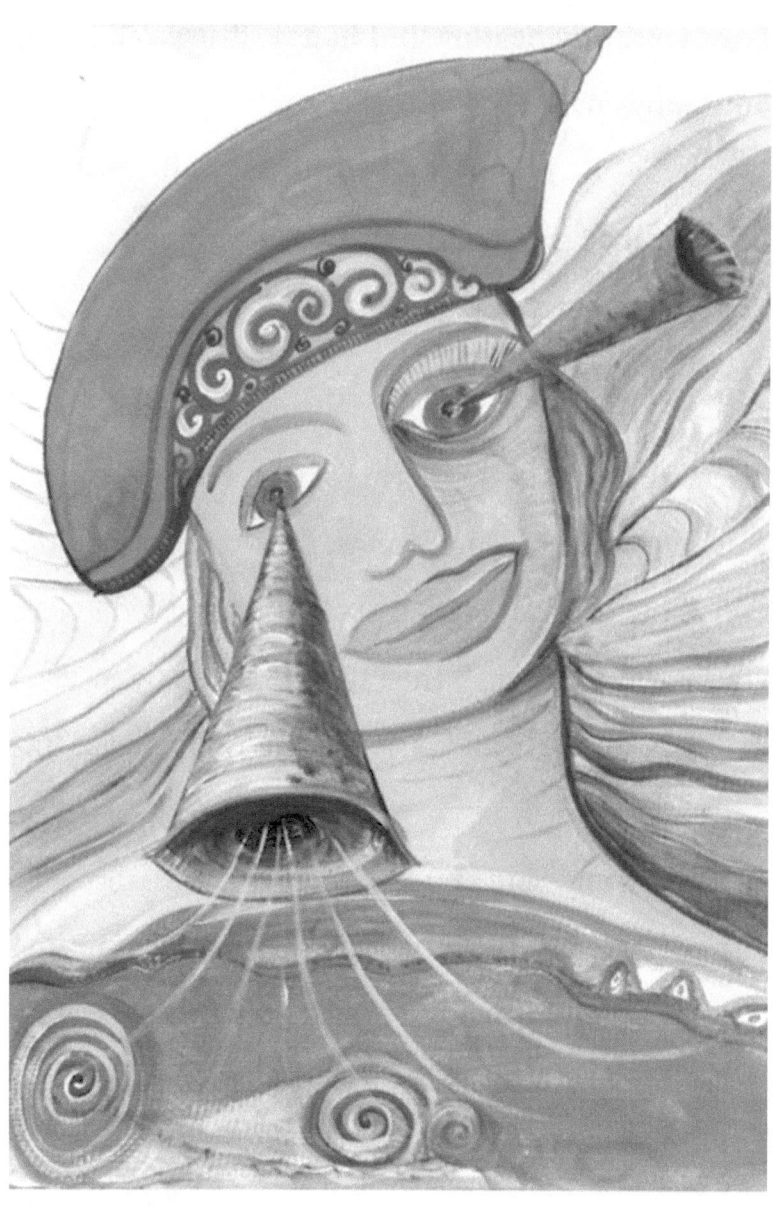

I am a beautiful person, a beautiful soul, and a beautiful spirit.

I am vibrantly healthy and happy. Every cell in my body sings with joy.

My baby is happy and healthy and growing beautifully. I give birth naturally and in joy.

My baby is born at the right time.

Every morning when Eternal and Soul awoke, they placed their hands on Eternal's belly and said, "I love you Forever, I love you Forever, I love you forever and ever." Soul caressed Eternal's belly and repeated, "I love you forever and ever." Then they wrapped themselves in a bubble of love and pure joy and wondered at this amazing experience.

Eternal and Soul affirmed these beautiful thoughts every day. Every time life hurt them, more amazing thoughts evolved, and they had a deep understanding that all people had been hurt just as they had been hurt.

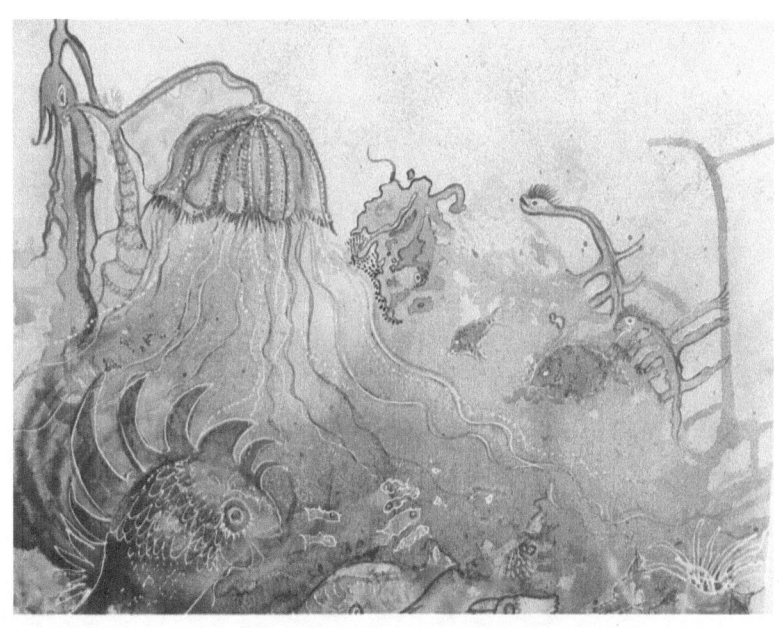

I love and respect people; people love and respect me.

I always bring the highest me to every circumstance I see.

Eternal and Soul were happy. Forever was growing beautifully, a precious bump forming in Eternal's belly.

Visualisation came as a wonderful gift and meditation to them both. Daily they used these gifts.

Chapter 5

Eternal and Soul searched books, the internet, and spoke to people, lapping up all the wisdom that they heard and read. They both found that they had begun to know the truth instinctively and intuitively wherever they found it.

They knew that every thought or deed, everything that Eternal ate, would impact Forever's physical health and mental well-being.

Each day was now a joyous time to rebirth and renew positive thought patterns and behaviours. Thoughts were shifting their wounded patterns, filtering out the old and replacing with the new. And they repeated the new thoughts over and over again.

Visualisation and meditation swept through them, cleansing and healing every cell in their bodies.

Eternal shared a visualisation with Soul.

She sat erect, her legs crossed, and took a series of long deep breaths. At times she found her mind wandering, and when it did, she brought the focus back to her breath, her life, and gently affirmed that she was a beautiful spirit, a beautiful soul, and a beautiful person whilst maintaining regular long deep breaths. She drifted into a beautiful place—her beautiful space—that, over time, she could choose to go to instantly and at any time.

Eternal was sitting on a mountain; a delightful warm breeze caressed her body. She could hear the birds singing and the bees buzzing, and there was a lovely fresh fragrance in the air. Eternal's body started to relax completely. She could feel Forever's presence with gentle movements.

Eternal walked along the mountain path in awe and wonder at God's creation, the myriad plants, flowers, trees, and creatures. She kept breathing deeply in a quiet rhythm. A butterfly darted to and fro. Then it flew down to her and landed on her shoulder. Eternal felt as if she was being cradled in God's warm caress. She had a deep understanding that we are truly all one.

Eternal saw a spiral whirling endlessly up into the sky. She was amazed as she saw millions of spirit humans as well as animals, fish, birds, and insects vibrating at different frequencies and with different levels of light emanating from them. Some of the humans she recognised.

They had held positions of great importance on Earth, wealthy, influential leaders of countries. But so too were there many ordinary people, and many of those ordinary people vibrated at the highest frequency and had the brightest light.

Eternal was conscious of everyone and each

expression, each movement. She breathed deeply and moved into the spiral, flowing along with it.

Some energies seemed to be hurrying along. They were being pushed to and fro. Frustration and anger radiated out of them as if they had grappled to reach life's pinnacle without searching for answers in life itself. The light they radiated was dim.

Some moved graciously, seemingly at peace with their lives. The light from them was strong and clear.

Eternal flowed on, breathing deeply. She became aware of how different the perception of the meaning and purpose of life was for each soul. In an instant, it was so clear. The most important things for all beings were the love and consciousness with which they lived their lives.

Eternal was entranced to be in the spiral, and she kept moving along, observing different faces—some in terrible pain, fear, and sadness; others showing serenity, peace, and love.

Eternity wanted to reach out to the entities, many of

them almost asleep and unconscious of who and what they were. She realised the highest gift is to understand that there is only this moment; live it consciously, love it consciously, so that each moment can be enjoyed, become a cherished memory, and create a fulfiled life. So that on reflection and in later years, we are at peace with how our life has been lived and the spirit, when it transcends this earthly plane, instantly becomes a part of God.

Eternal understood that each being on the spiral had endeavoured to be the best he or she could be relative to the evolution of one's soul. Eternal resolved to do all she could to help Forever be the brightest energy imaginable.

Eternal was given the greatest gift she could imagine. As she drifted within the spiral, she began to feel infused with the love and power of every woman who had ever given birth, filling her with the strength for the birth that lay ahead.

Gradually, Eternal's energy moved down, back into her body, to Forever growing in her belly, and she visualised a wonderful birth and life with Forever and Soul.

Chapter 6

Eternal's pregnancy had been uneventful. They had wanted to have a baby at the right time, and Forever had decided it was the right time. Tests confirmed Forever's presence, and Eternal and Soul were so excited.

Life went on, and Eternal and Soul did what they always did, thought good thoughts, but they still rushed to work, grabbed hurried meals, and occasionally partied. This pregnancy wouldn't change their lifestyle!

Eternal awoke from a beautiful sleep, unaware of

the sadness that was to unfold. It was the weekend, and Soul was already up and working in the garden. The sun was streaming in through the bedroom window. Eternal reached down to feel the reassuring movements of Forever growing inside her.

She caressed her belly gently and waited. No response. She caressed her belly again. Still no response. Panic arose as Eternal called out to Soul, for him to reassure her. She knew she had felt less movement in the last few days. If she could just feel one more movement. Eternal had spent yesterday hoping to feel more movement, but there had been little.

Eternal's belly was still. There was no sign of Forever's life. Tears flowed down Eternal's cheeks like a torrent as she feared the worst. Eternal and Soul drove to get help, but sadly, their worst fears were confirmed.

Forever had chosen to go home. Why?

What had Eternal done to deserve this? She was a good person. Was it something she had done?

- Did she really want a baby?

- Was it something she had eaten?

- Was it that she had been so busy, or was it that she had slipped whilst in a hurry? Was it her fault?

- Or was it the tablets she had taken when she was not feeling well?

- Yes, she had a few drinks.

- She had smoked just a few cigarettes a day. (Smoking can do you *no* good; it can only do you and your baby harm.)

Tests revealed nothing wrong with Forever.

When a soul knows that the material body has not formed properly or has a condition not compatible with its life, this incarnation, and the lessons it seeks to learn, it will sometimes decide to go home.

Forever birthed some days later with the help of some angels in human form.

His little body perfect, the memory of his tiny

little hands and toes and soft body were etched into Eternal's and Soul's very beings.

Eternal swept him up and held him so close, as if to breathe life into him or to feel one last movement. Soul wrapped his arms around them both as they grieved together, loving Forever and longing for what might have been.

They held on to his perfect little body, not bearing to part with him. But eventually, they took Forever's little body and gave him back to the earth. They planted a beautiful tree in his memory. Eternal's and Soul's tears rolled uncontrollably down their cheeks.

Forever will always be in their hearts. A beautiful framed picture of his footprint and handprint are the only lasting material memory of this little soul.

Grief turned to surrender as Eternal and Soul felt the pain of Forever's loss. They believed that one day they would again be with Forever.

1. If you have decreased movement, contact the hospital to check all is well. Heazell, A. (2012). Reduced fetal movements. *BMC Pregnancy Childbirth*, *12*(Suppl 1), A10. http://dx.doi.org/10.1186/1471-2393-12-s1-a10Heazell, A. (2015). A kick in the right direction—reduced fetal movements and stillbirth prevention. *BMC Pregnancy Childbirth*, *15*(Suppl 1), A7. http://dx.doi.org/10.1186/1471-2393-15-s1-a7.

2. Safe foods in pregnancy booklet. Stone, J., Eddleman, K., & Duenwald, M. (2009). *Pregnancy for Dummies*. Hoboken, NJ: John Wiley & Sons.

3. Never take any medication without confirming it is safe during pregnancy. Christopher, L. (2008). Taking Drugs during Pregnancy. *Developmental Medicine & Child Neurology*, *20*(3), 380–383. http://dx.doi.org/10.1111/j.1469-8749.1978.tb15229.x.

4. There is no safe level of alcohol intake during pregnancy according to the WHO. Alcohol consumption during pregnancy. (2016). April 1, 2016, from http://World Health Organisation on Alcohol during pregnancy.

5. Smoking can do you no good; it can only do you and your baby harm. Oaks, L. (2001). *Smoking and Pregnancy.* New Brunswick, NJ: Rutgers University Press.

6. Crying is good for healing. Scientists have found the chemical makeup of tears from grief and stress are different from reflexive tears. Brody, J. (1982). *Biological Role of Emotional Tears.* Retrieved August 16, 2016, from http://www. nytimes.com 1982/08/31science.

7. There is healing in talking. Harding, G. (2005). *Surviving in the Hour of Darkness.* Calgary, AB: University of Calgary Press.

Chapter 7

Grief and sadness were etched into their souls. Why did Forever abandon them when he was so loved? They had told him so every day. And with every thought, they had done everything possible to ensure Eternal was in vibrant health both mentally and physically. Disbelief shrouded their minds.

Soul went into his cave and spoke very little. Anger covered his sadness. This was somehow acceptable for a man; it was how he could deal with his sense of helplessness.

Eternal wept uncontrollably, longing for what

might have been, wondering how she could ever face the world again.

Facing each day with optimism and faith would be the ultimate challenge for them, knowing that it is not what happens but, rather, the way it is handled. For some reason, Forever was unable to stay on Earth this time.

Eternal's grief lingered for months. Each day it was an effort to get out of bed. She felt as if she had been kicked in the pit of her stomach and had swallowed acid that was slowly eating away at her insides. Eternal knew that now, more than ever, she needed to be gentle with herself and maintain her prayers, meditations, and affirmations.

Eternal retraced her steps again and again. What could she have done differently? What had she done wrong? She longed to feel at peace again.

Sadly, many of her dear friends chose not to talk about her loss. Rather, they gave them sympathy cards with meaningless words and pictures of flowers. How would that help with their desperate feelings?

Eternal knew they meant well, and for them, it was just too painful or embarrassing to talk about death. We know we are born and that death is a given. But still, we find it hard to accept. Eternal longed for them to acknowledge the loss and just talk about how they were feeling.

Making love with Soul felt empty. But Eternal's rising thoughts of not being good enough to be a mother were quickly countered with loving affirmations.

I love myself, I love myself, I am love

Soul felt he had let down Eternal. Yet he took comfort in knowing they had done all they could to become the best parents.

Eventually, a new day dawned for Eternal and Soul. They both knew the spirit that was Forever would return someday.

Eternal awoke feeling strong and vibrant for the

first time since Forever's return home. Her thoughts turned inward, and she felt blessed. She felt Forever's presence and energy, and gave thanks for the gift of peace she was feeling again.

Yet she also had a slight queasy feeling in her stomach.

Could she be?

Maybe she was!

Yes! She knew without a doubt that Forever, that beautiful soul, was returning to them.

Affirmations for Pregnancy/Birth

I love myself.

I welcome with great joy this soul that has chosen me.

I meditate, visualise, and affirm the perfect birth.

I am conscious of every thought I have, and I choose only the good.

Every cell in my body vibrates with love, joy, health, and abundance.

I draw the right people into my life to support me during my pregnancy and the birth of my baby.

I love my pregnant body.

My baby is growing perfectly.

I feel wonderfully happy, healthy, and strong.

I trust my body to support my pregnancy and the birth.

People love and support me.

My partner loves and supports me.

I am totally serene and calm.

Birthing Affirmations

My higher power is with me at all times, guiding and directing my life.

I affirm drawing in good at all times.

I trust my body.

My body knows how to give birth gently.

I draw on all the women who have given birth for their strength, love, and power.

I am vibrantly heathy and ready to birth my baby into the world.

I draw the right people into my life for the best birth.

I am completely relaxed and visualise my baby moving effortlessly through the birth canal.

I breathe deeply in a flowing, calming rhythm.

With each event (contraction), I relax completely.

I relax my face, my forehead, my lips, my shoulders, my arms, and my whole body.

My cervix softens and dilates effortlessly.

My perineum is soft and pliable.

My uterus pushes my baby gently into the world.

My uterus contacts and expels the placenta at the right time.

My baby crawls up to my breast to suckle.

About the Author

I am Mary Anne Howard-Clarke, RN RM-eligible midwife, educator, and speaker. My life's purpose is primarily a spiritual one, to serve my fellow human beings. As a young child at boarding school in Africa, I had an extraordinary dream and a vision of the important healing path that lay ahead for me. I have been so privileged to have been part of many people's lives as they faced some of their most challenging times.

I was born on a farm in Donkerhoek in what was then the Eastern Transvaal of South Africa. My grandmother delivered me, and I was always fascinated that she was so calm and matter of fact as she talked about the babies she had delivered as she had no formal midwifery training! This sparked my fascination with birth, and I spent many hours watching the farm animals give birth. Initially I wanted to help animals and become a veterinary nurse. The sad truth is that animals cannot talk and tell you what is wrong with them, and this understanding was a pivotal moment that led me in a different direction. I decided to become a nurse and midwife.

I trained in London. I took my general training at St Marys Hospital, Paddington, and my midwifery at Queen Charlottes Maternity Hospital.

Since qualifying, I have worked in many countries— the United Kingdom, South Africa, Swaziland, New Zealand, and since the early 2000s, Australia. I have enjoyed working in both remote and rural environments, as well as large centres. It has been my absolute privilege to have shared the journey of many people as they both enter and leave this life.

I presently work at the Mater Hospital in the Redlands, near Brisbane, as a nurse and midwife. I also run my own practice, Ask the Midwife, which offers postnatal services and home assistance.

I also married and had four wonderful children. I have seven grandchildren and live on the Brisbane Bayside in Queensland, Australia.